BODY BASICS
fore golfers

Stay in the game,
avoid pain!

Here's what people are saying about
BODY BASICS *fore golfers*

"A simple and easy-to-use guide to ensure a healthy and safe approach to the game."
JAN LOWTHER RN. COHN(C)

"As an orthopaedic surgeon and avid golfer, I recognize that fitness is an all too often neglected part of this great sport. Finally, an easy to read, sensible book, specifically written with the golfer in mind. Karen Webb should be commended for putting together Body Basics fore golfers, which without doubt, will allow golfers of all ages to avoid pain and stay in the game!"
RALPH POTOTSCHNIK M.D.. FRCS(C)
ORTHOPAEDIC SURGEON

"An excellent practical book that all golfers need. Keep it in your golf bag along with your rules book. Make it your goal to finish every round of golf pain-free by simple year round attention to your posture, flexibility and strength. Find out what you can do with the most important piece of golf equipment, your body, to lower your score."
LINDA MCLAREN B.S.R.
PHYSICAL THERAPIST. BRITISH COLUMBIA

"Healthy living, and the game of golf — two of life's pleasures! This book teaches us just how simple it can be to enjoy both. A must read for any golfer."
KERRY PRICE B.SC.H.K.
HEART HEALTH PERTH COORDINATOR. FORMER YMCA LIFESTYLE DIRECTOR

"As is appropriate and supported by the scientific literature, this book demonstrates in a practical manner, how spinal health and injury prevention is attainable to all, through postural habits and lifestyle choices."
IONE PUCHALSKI D.C.. CCRD.DAC BOH
CHIROPRACTOR

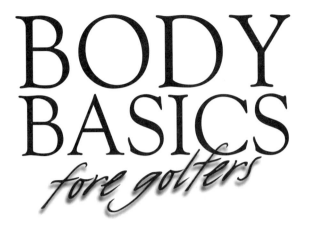

BODY BASICS
fore golfers

Stay in the game,
avoid pain!

Karen Webb
B.P.T., MCPA

Birchcliff Publishing Inc.
Stratford, Ontario, Canada

Copyright © 1999 by Birchcliff Publishing Inc.

All rights reserved. No part of this publication may be reproduced, stored in a retrieval system, or transmitted, in any form or by any means, without the prior written permission of the copyright owner, except by a reviewer who may quote brief passages in a review.

Body Basics *for life* is a trademark of Birchcliff Publishing Inc.

Canadian Cataloguing in Publication Data.

Webb, Karen, 1953–
  Body Basics *fore golfers:* stay in the game, avoid pain!

Includes bibliographical references.
ISBN 0-9682571-2-7

1. Golf-Training.	2. Golf injuries-Prevention.	I. Title.
II. Title: Body basics.	II. Body basics for golfers	
RC 1220.G64 W42 1999	613.7'11	C98-901312-X

Production Art by Garratt Graphics.
Photography by Michael McClintock.
Editing by Layne Verbeek.
Cover & Author Photo by Elisabeth Feryn.
Bench Prop on Cover: property Johnny's Antiques, Shakespeare, Ontario, Canada.
Golf Props on Cover: property of David Lee, C.P.G.A. Professional, Pro Shop, The Stratford Country Club.
Printed in Canada by The Beacon Herald Fine Printing Division, Stratford, Ontario.

All inquiries should be addressed to:
Birchcliff Publishing Inc.
Suite 126, 59 Albert Street
Stratford, Ontario
Canada N5A 3K2
(519) 273-3334
E-mail: birchclf@orc.ca

Quantity discounts are available on bulk purchases of this book. For information contact Birchcliff Publishing Inc. at the above address or call us at (519) 273-3334 or toll free at 1-888-472-9121.
A mail-order form is located in the back of the book.

Body Basics *fore golfers*: Stay in the game, avoid pain! is not intended as medical advice. This book's intention is solely educational and informational while lending itself to prevention and self-help. The reader should regularly consult a physician in matters relating to his or her health and individual needs. Clearance from your physician is recommended prior to beginning an exercise program. The author and the publisher expressly disclaim any liability, loss, or risk, personal or otherwise, which is incurred as a consequence, directly or indirectly, of the use and application of any of the contents of this book.

To golfers of all ages: there will often be obstacles in our lives that prevent us from playing — pain should not be one of these!

ACKNOWLEDGEMENTS

Production Art by Garratt Graphics

Photography by Michael McClintock

Editing by Layne Verbeek

Cover & Author Photograph by Elisabeth Feryn

Cover bench prop courtesy of Johnny's Antiques

Cover golf props courtesy of David Lee, Pro,
The Stratford Country Club

Paul, Samantha and Kirstie Webb, have always been there for me when I needed them. I thank them for this and equally important, I thank them for knowing when not to be there.

David Lee is a C.P.G.A. Golf Pro at the Stratford Country Club. David generously provided golf equipment for the book cover photo, and he has been instrumental in the successful photo sessions at the golf course. Although I can't necessarily give David credit for the weather that allowed many of us to golf right into December 1998.

Both an ergonomic consultant and a golfer, I met Kevin Schouppe at a 1998 conference for workplace injury prevention. Kevin's keen interest and research in the biomechanics of the golf swing motivated me to pursue this project and he has always been helpful and just a quick e-mail away.

Dianne Zakaria is a physiotherapist and is completing her doctorate program. Dianne has always been willing to help out and provide constructive suggestions. Once again, I appreciate her support on this project.

I want to thank the staff of the Stratford Public Library for their continuing help in my research efforts.

And my sincere thanks goes out to all the models appearing in this book, and as the old saying goes, a picture is worth a thousand words.

CONTENTS

KEEP YOUR BODY
UP TO PAR

Enjoy Golf? Looking forward to spending more time on your favorite course? Then this is the book for you.

As a golfer, your body is very important to you. Yet most people don't realize the impact that everyday living has on their bodies — nor how this can affect their golf game. We place a tremendous amount of physical strain on ourselves from prolonged sitting, repetitive movements and poor standing and resting habits. Their long-term effects develop innocently, are often overlooked, but then become chronic — even severe enough to take you out of the game.

As a physiotherapist with more than twenty years' experience, I have treated many golfers. And, the physical complaints of many of these golfers were often preventable. Most of their problems were either lifestyle related or resulted from improper warm-ups or lack of conditioning. With our aging population, increased spare time, and a growing interest in golf, I expect the number of golfers seeking assistance from health professionals to dramatically increase over the next few years.

This book is subtitled *Stay in the game, avoid pain!* because that's what I promise to teach you. The simple tasks in this book will make it easy for you to understand the causes of unnecessary body pain as well as how to avoid them both on and off the golf course.

If pain hasn't prevented you from enjoying your game, chances are it will at some point in the future. Back pain alone affects eight out of ten of us at some time in our lives and, next to the common cold, it is the most frequent complaint we bring to our doctors. In most cases of physical complaints, the pain could have been avoided if the person had the right information or know-how to prevent it. The basic lessons in this book will help you solve many postural complaints, as well as help you prevent injuries and other health problems from ever starting.

As a golfer, your body is very important to you. Yet most people don't realize the impact everyday living has on their bodies.

KEEP YOUR BODY
UP TO PAR

As you will see, I've provided lots of practical information with helpful photographs in this book. It covers a variety of golf-specific topics which include pre-season preparation, game warm-up and cool-down, golfers' feet, and healthy habits for the golf course. I have also included tips for carrying golf bags and other carry items.

This book also explains how you can avoid muscular problems that result from repetitive activities. It describes good sitting and standing postures as well as survival exercises for your neck and back. And finally, it provides tips on how you can stay fit for golf all year round.

Time constraints may prevent you from playing golf as often as you would like — but pain and lack of physical well being should not! These healthy habits and exercises will start you on the way to a happy and pain-free life — *and* give you more time on the golf course.

Karen Webb

GOLFERS OF ALL AGES, THROUGH THE AGES

There are differing opinions on the origins of the game of golf. Its roots can be traced back to at least the mid-1400s. Scotland is recognized as being the home of St. Andrews, the world's oldest golf course, and Canada is credited with having the first permanent course in North America, the Royal Montreal Club founded in 1873. And one of the older American clubs, also named St. Andrews, was established in 1888 in Yonkers, New York.

While there may be some question as to the origin of golf, there is no question as to its growing popularity in North America and around the world. Once dominated by men and recognized as an activity of the well-to-do, the game is becoming increasingly popular with women, children, and people from all walks of life. Younger, high profile professional players have captured our children's attention and this has caused junior golf camps and clinics to spring up across the country. At the same time, the large number of baby boomers, with decreasing family and work commitments, are finding more time to spend on the course.

Unlike many other sports, golf can be a life-long pleasure.

Unlike many other sports, golf can be a life-long pleasure. And it can be started at an early age and enjoyed throughout one's senior years.

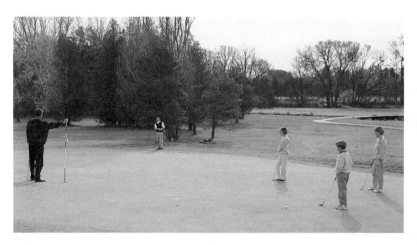

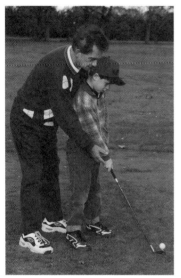

For the older golfer who wants to spend more time on the course and play well into his or her senior years, it is important that he or she understands a number of physical aspects related to older age. They need to understand the natural aging process of their bodies; the impact their lifestyle is having on their physical well being; and what simple steps they can take to avoid and prevent unnecessary pain and injury. By understanding your body and following these simple steps, you will not only be physically and mentally better but will also enjoy improvement in your game.

Although the physical *aspects* of the game are also important for children, they are not as critical as golf safety aspects. Children rarely have serious aches and pains with golf because they are more active, have greater flexibility, and bend instinctively long before they develop poor physical habits. But while they are developing their golf skills, learning rules of play and understanding golf etiquette, children also need to be aware of the physical *dangers* that they may face. Therefore, knowing where to stand while other players hit the ball; ensuring a safe distance between themselves and other groups on the course; and the dangers associated with water hazards; lightning; excess exposure to the sun; and unfamiliar vegetation all become things to watch out for.

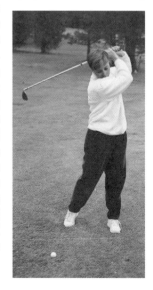

BENDING

Your spine consists of your neck, mid-back, low back, sacrum (triangular bone below your low back) and tail bone. Jelly doughnut-like discs separate the bones in your neck, mid-back and low back allowing for movement. The neck has a tremendous amount of rotation, allowing you to safely look over your shoulder when driving a car, riding a bike or teeing off. Rotation in your lower back is small and this is why we hear about lower back twisting type injuries.

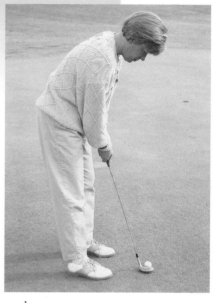

One big mistake we tend to make is that we do not keep our necks and lower backs mobile. We tend to move our spine repeatedly in one direction but seldomly in the opposite direction. The most common excess movement we do in our lower back is forward bending, such as tying a shoe or sitting in a chair. And, the most common excess movements in our neck are forward bending combined with a poking of our heads forward. As a physiotherapist, I saw many people with conditions developing from excess movement that they could have prevented. The movements we must also do regularly are backward bending of our lower backs and backward bending of our necks.

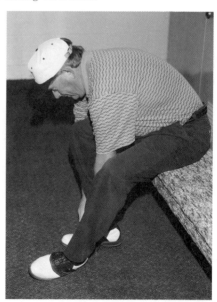

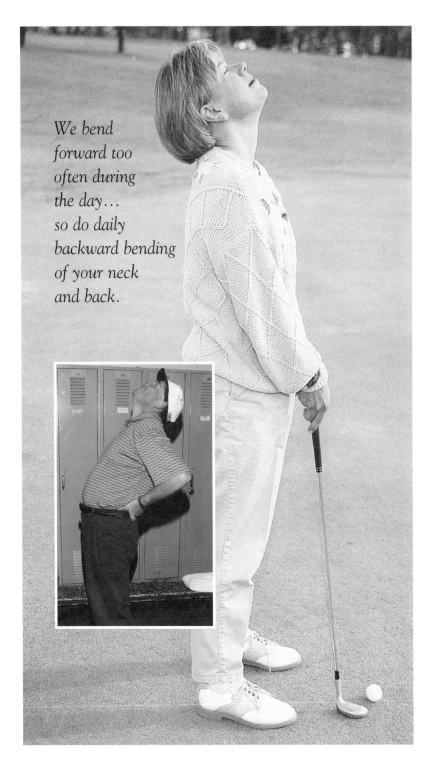

We bend forward too often during the day… so do daily backward bending of your neck and back.

13

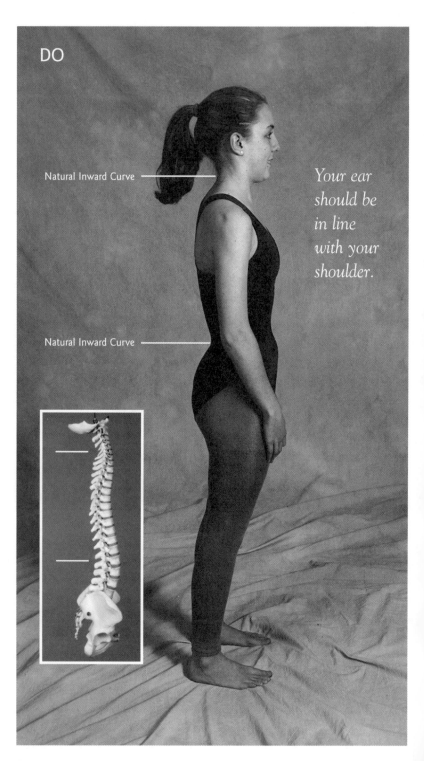

DO

Natural Inward Curve ————

Natural Inward Curve ————

Your ear should be in line with your shoulder.

POSTURES FOR LIFE ARE POSTURES FOR GOLF

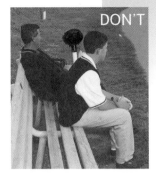

DON'T

It is important to remember that your posture off the course can greatly affect your play on the course. For golf is like any other sport — it makes extra demands on many parts of your body. Athletes know that they must take proper body care in all aspects of their life to perform well in their sport. This is the same for golf.

Your neck has a natural inward curve or hollow just above your shoulders. When standing upright, your ears should line with your shoulders. Postural pain results from not paying attention or not knowing how to sit or stand. People most often get these problems from carrying their heads in front of their bodies with their chins poking forward.

Poor posture over the long term can be just as harmful as an injury.

Your lower back also has a natural inward curve, or hollow. This hollow is lost when your lower back is rounded from a poor sitting posture or when you are bent forward.

Robin McKenzie, an internationally respected physiotherapist from New Zealand, is recognized as an expert in neck and back pain. He believes poor posture over the long term can be just as harmful as an injury. He also believes most deformities in the elderly are the visible effects of long-standing poor posture habits and are, more importantly, preventable. I agree with Robin McKenzie's statement in his book Treat Your Own Back, "...spinal pain of a postural origin would not occur if basic education were given to individuals at an early age."

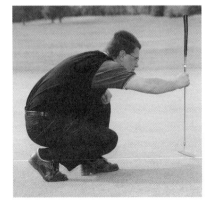

As a golfer, good posture is important in order to correctly address the golf ball. Our everyday activities, such as prolonged sitting, driving or gardening challenge us. Remember to maintain a natural, healthy spinal curve.

SITTING

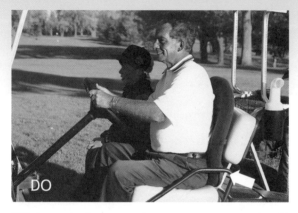

DO

While we don't necessarily associate sitting with golf — sitting certainly does come into play. Unless you have the luxury of living in a condominium next to a golf course, you will start your day by sitting in your car to drive to the course. On a busy day, you may also be faced with a long wait for your turn to tee off. And after all this, you will probably find yourself sitting again at the 19th hole at the end of the day!

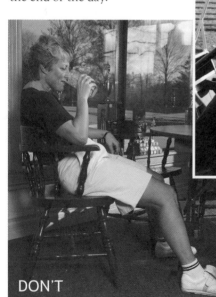

DON'T

DON'T

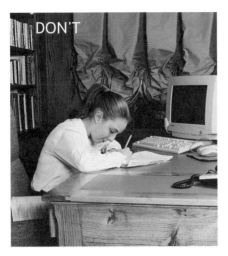

DON'T

Pay attention to how you sit, for we often sit for long periods of time in harmful positions and poor posture. Some of us sit forward on the edge of our chair, hunched over with our heads buried in a book. Some lean on one elbow creating a sideward curve in their spine. And, some of us have our arms held out, unsupported, while typing. All of these activities lead to the same result — sore necks, backs and shoulders, and sometimes headaches.

When you sit, the muscles supporting your lower back get tired. And with muscle fatigue, the inward curve, or hollow, in your lower back is lost and you slouch. Muscles that support your head and neck also tire and the inward curve in your neck is lost leaving your head and neck to poke forward. And once the slouch in your lower back takes over, it is next to impossible to maintain good posture of your head and neck.

Practice:
Learn to feel
the difference
between good
and bad.

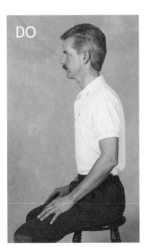

DO

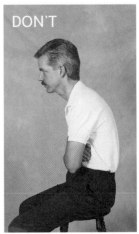

DON'T

SITTING

You should avoid sitting without a backrest for long periods of time. A slouching posture will slowly take over no matter how hard you try to avoid it. Some chairs do provide good support to our lower backs but most do not. We have to be prepared to add our own lower back support.

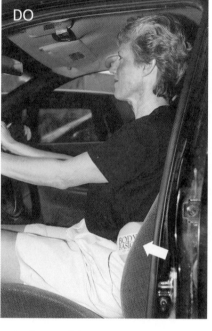

I take my lower back roll everywhere. It can be used in any chair, sofa, car or restaurant seat. Just simply place the roll in the small of your back at your waistline. If you drive a lot, keep a roll in your car for extra support. You can also use full back supports for this.

You should also pay particular attention to the posture of your "little" golfers. Children sit for hours in front of the television, video games and computers, and are now developing poor posture and pain at earlier ages. To

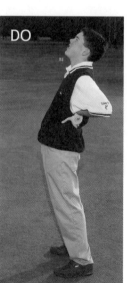

avoid this, get them to take breaks and move around every half hour. They should also do simple stretching exercises that take barely a minute to perform.

Dominated by sitting and forward bending, our lifestyle is taking its toll on golfers.

Healthy Hints

User friendly
desk work:

• Stretch arms,
hands, neck
and back every
60 minutes or
sooner if you
feel a strain

• Walk around
every once in
awhile

• If you use the
phone often,
try to get a
hands-free
headset or
speaker phone

SEATING

• If your chair doesn't have adequate support, use a back roll, back support, or rolled up towel to support the inward curve in your lower back
• Keep your feet flat on a foot rest or flat on the floor

KEYBOARDING

• Keep your shoulders relaxed and your arms at the sides of your body
• Keep your elbows bent at 90°
• Hold your forearms and wrists parallel to the floor

SCREEN

• Sit about one arm's length back from the screen
• Position your monitor so the top line of print is level with your eyes
• Keep your head and neck upright

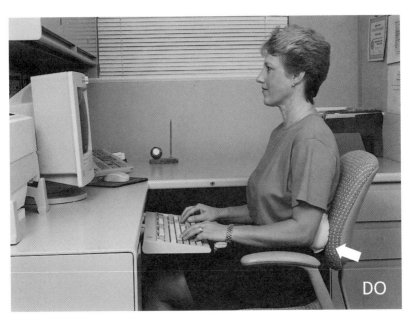

DO

SURVIVAL EXERCISES

'SLOPPY' PUSH-UP

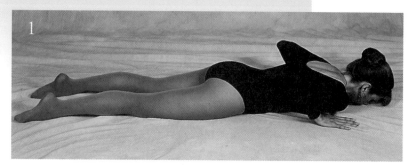

1. Lie face down and place your hands under your shoulders

2. Straighten your elbows and allow your back to sag.
   Hold this for two counts

Repeat this exercise five to ten times

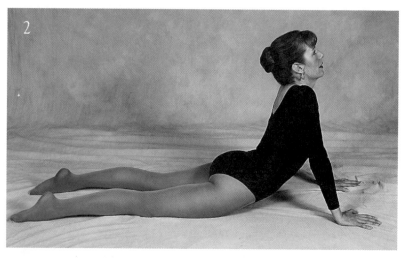

Healthy Hints

Do 'sloppy' push-ups:

• As part of your morning routine

• As part of your night routine

• Before and after every abdominal muscle
  workout

BACK BEND

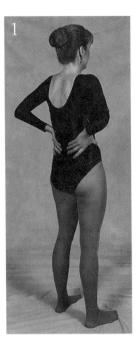

1. While standing, place your hands in the small of your back, with your fingers pointing inwards

2. Bend backwards at your waist keeping your knees straight. Hold this for two counts

Repeat this exercise five times

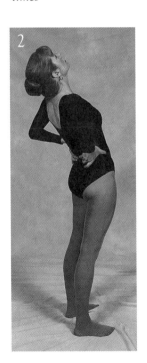

Healthy Hints

Do back bends:

• Prior to lifting your golf bag out of your car

• Prior to every game of golf (during and after as needed)

• Prior to, and during repeated lifting

• While sitting for long periods of time

• Following every strenuous workout

• When you feel minor strains developing in your back on or off the golf course

CHIN TUCK

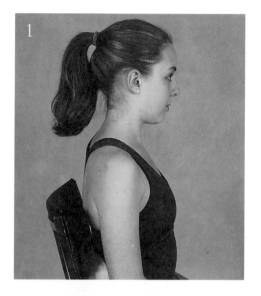

1. Sit with good back posture. Look straight ahead and relax

2. Move your head straight back with your eyes looking forward. Imagine you have a plate of peas on top of your head that you don't want to spill. Hold this for two counts

Repeat this exercise five times

Healthy Hints

Do chin tucks:

• As part of your morning routine

• As part of your night routine

• While doing desk work for long periods of time

• After every strenuous workout

• After every abdominal muscle workout that strains your neck

• When you feel minor strains developing in your neck

• As part of your cool down after your golf game

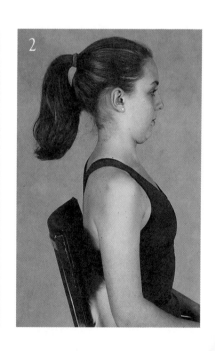

BACKWARD NECK BEND

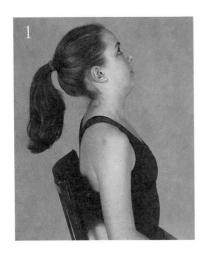

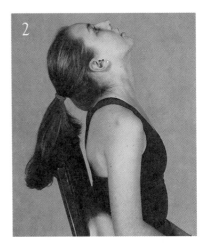

1. While holding your 'chin tuck', tilt your head backwards

2. Let go of your chin tuck to allow you to move your head back as far as comfortably possible. Hold this for two counts

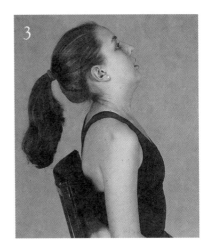

3. As you bring your head up, regain your chin tuck and then return to an upright position

Repeat this exercise five times

Healthy Hints

Do backward neck bends:

- Prior to, during and after every game of golf

- While doing desk work for long periods of time

- After every abdominal muscle workout that strains your neck

- After sleeping on your stomach

FIT FOR GOLF

FITNESS

A person's level of fitness does not stay constant. It changes in response to a number of factors, many of which we can either control or learn to control. Some of these factors include good posture, proper exercise, adequate rest, and proper diet and weight control. Fit people avoid excessive drinking. They also avoid smoking and using drugs. Getting proper medical care is also important. But, bear in mind that ignoring one area of your body's health can affect the good things you do for another part of your body. A diet aimed at weight loss and improved body composition must also include an exercise plan.

Numerous health risks are associated with excess body fat. Heart disease tops the list. In North America more people are overweight today than ten years ago — and this includes children.

Basic nutrition is important. We need foods from each of the four basic food groups. Make plant foods, such as cereal, grains, vegetables and fruit the cornerstones of your diet. But don't make the mistake of increasing your portions just because you're eating healthy foods. Excess carbohydrates such as breads are also extra calories that will be stored as fat. Eat moderate amounts of low fat foods from the milk and meat groups. Finally, go sparingly on fats, oils, and sweets.

Always take a bottle of water and a healthy snack in your golf bag.

Make good choices. Choose a manual golf cart over an electric golf cart. If carrying your clubs, use a two strap system. Choose stairs over an elevator. Walk or cycle to the store instead of driving. Park your car some distance from the shopping mall entrance. Spend time with your family during evenings or weekends. Keep on the move and try new things. The more physically fit you are, the better your body can handle both physical and emotional stress.

So, as a fit golfer, you are less likely to injure yourself during the game — and it will take a lot more to get your blood pressure to rise.

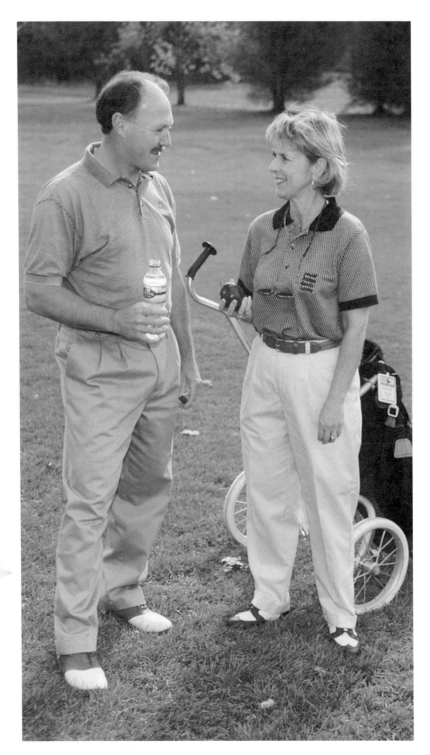

FIT FOR GOLF

WHY WE NEED TO EXERCISE

1. BODY COMPOSITION

Body composition refers to the percentage of body fat compared to lean tissue. Percentage of body fat increases with normal aging. This increase is caused by changes in our bodies' basal metabolic rate (rate at which the body uses energy to maintain itself during complete rest) and reduced physical activity. Our bodies adapt to specific physical demands placed on them. If we exercise, our bodies meet the demand. And, if we exercise regularly, we experience good long-term effects and our bodies become leaner.

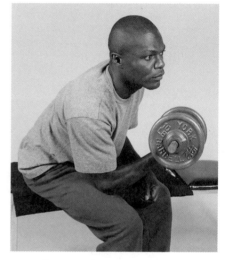

2. MUSCLE

Muscle mass naturally starts to decline as early as age 30. It is believed that after age 40, most women lose nearly one quarter of a kilogram (half a pound) of muscle each year. Research proves that strengthening exercises reverse this decline. Muscle strength and endurance is important to your golf game.

With strength training, your muscles develop more tiny blood vessels. These new capillaries deliver nutrients and oxygen to the muscle fibers and get rid of waste products. This all helps you prevent injuries on and off the golf course.

3. FLEXIBILITY

Tissues connecting bones together at our joints become stiffer as we age. This reduced flexibility is linked to reduced activity and can also be improved through exercise with a stretching program. Reduced flexibility can lead to pain, and on the course it can adversely affect your golf swing.

Don't forget your most important piece of golf equipment is your body — exercise it regularly.

4. BONES

Osteoporosis (thinning bones) concerns everyone. Bones become thinner as we age. Weight bearing exercises such as walking, jogging, and resistive exercises (weight training) are proven to help maintain bone thickness or density. A proper diet and a regular exercise program needs to be introduced early in life to help prevent such problems.

5. HEART RATE

Your heart is also a muscle and needs to be worked. Our maximum heart rate declines with age. The amount of blood pumped out of the heart per beat increases with exercise and overcomes the effect of a lowered maximum heart rate.

6. OXYGEN UPTAKE

Maximum oxygen uptake (bringing in and using oxygen) declines after the age of 30. Our body's ability to bring in and use oxygen improves with exercise training at any age, and is especially important as we get older. The harder you work these systems, the better and the longer these systems work for you.

7. NATURAL PAINKILLERS

Your brain produces natural painkillers called endorphins. If you exercise regularly, your body will produce more of these chemicals. Endorphins are responsible for that feeling of extreme well being, common amongst runners after their workout.

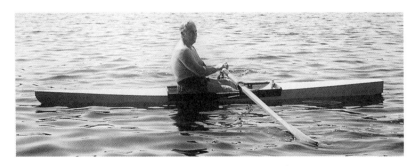

TIRED MUSCLES

BODY BASICS for golfers

ARM YOURSELF AGAINST
UPPER BODY ABUSE

We tend to take our arms and hands for granted. Yet our fingers, hands, wrists, elbows, and shoulders are all capable of a great deal of skill and grace. We can sew a button on a shirt, pick a crumb up off the table or turn a page in a book. We can cast a fishing line, play table tennis or turn a skipping rope. More importantly, as golfers, we can drive a golf ball a few hundred yards, and we can putt with fine tuned precision. Our muscles work best when they are moving.

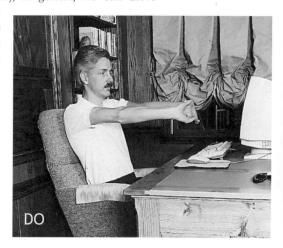

DO

Healthy Hints

- Take a break from your activity and stretch every hour. The more intensive the activity, the more frequently you need to break

- If you feel a strain in your neck, arms or back: Stop and stretch! Mini breaks are sometimes needed

- Pace yourself with every project. Give your body parts a break when doing things like painting a fence, raking leaves or doing a puzzle

- Remember to *stretch* your eyes and periodically look away from your television or computer

- Listen to your body. Pain is its warning signal

- Make sure your golf routines and playing schedules have an adequate amount of time in between for rest and recovery

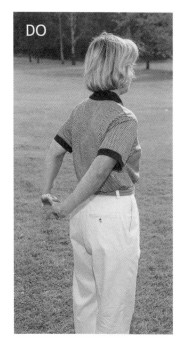

DO

When you make your muscles work without movement, such as holding a sign above your head for several minutes, the blood supply to your muscles slows down. If you work at a keyboard for an hour, your muscles get tired and achy. Stress is placed on the nerves and blood vessels that run down the length of your arm. These get bent at your elbow just like a kink in a garden hose, interrupting the natural flow. Leaving these nerves bent for long periods of time can lead to painful problems.

The second harmful habit is when you perform repeated movements over long periods of time. This is how repetitive strain injuries develop. We don't realize what we are asking of these small muscles and joints when we intensively knit, type or play the piano.

Our arms are stronger in one direction of movement because of our regular and repeated daily activities. These muscles are the muscles that allow us to grip the handle of a suitcase or to hug someone. At the same time, the muscles that move our arms in the opposite direction are normally weaker since we use them less. These weaker muscles, some of which are important to your golf swing, are more vulnerable to injury.

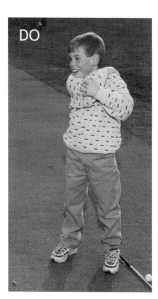

DO

Listen to your body. Pain is its warning signal.

YEAR ROUND CONDITIONING

Are you one of those enthusiastic golfers who plays 18 holes on the first warm day of spring, and then suffers? If so, you are not alone. Unconditioned bodies are always at risk for injury both on and off the golf course. Even if you stretched before the game, a few minutes of stretching is not enough.

Year round conditioning is your ticket to improved energy and well being both on and off the golf course. If you are fit and your body is well tuned, you will handle stress in stride, avoid unnecessary pain and injuries, and your golf game will improve. Using the best golf equipment will not lower your score or prevent injuries. You need flexibility, strength and endurance to do that. Your body is your most important piece of golf equipment and it must be cared for well.

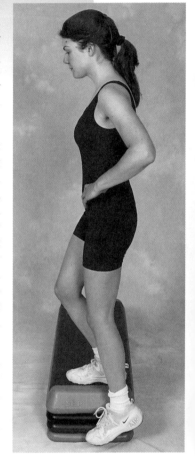

A year-round conditioning program should consist of strengthening exercises, stretching exercises, and activity for your heart and lungs. But remember to start off slowly and gradually increase the intensity of your program.

The exercises listed here will provide you with a good basic routine. The strengthening component addresses a number of general muscle groups as well as specific muscle groups used in the golf swing. Strengthening helps prevent injuries, improve joint stability and results in a smooth and efficient swing. Specific exercises for the forearm, wrist and hand are covered in the Pre-Season Preparation section. And, remember to consult a golf professional to ensure good technique.

Experts now know that not only do we lose muscle mass at an early age but that we can also work to reverse this process. The great thing about strength training is that you reap its benefits long after your workout ends.

Always remember to warm your muscles before stretching or strength training. You can do this passively by taking a shower or actively by moving your legs and arms. A few minutes of walking, jumping jacks, or jogging on the spot will also help you warm your muscles easily.

Work on developing your muscle strength first; then focus on muscular endurance. (Muscle strength is the power that your muscles have and muscle endurance is the ability for your muscles to work for long periods of time without fatigue.)

You can do weight training in your home or at a gym. While free weights, dumb bells and exercise machines work well, you can also use your own body weight as resistance (such as push-ups, crunches or squats). Other weight training tools can include soup cans, books, and specialty strengthening bands.

If you lack flexibility, strength and endurance, even the best equipment will not help you lower your score or prevent injuries.

However, weight training and resistive exercises should not be done daily. For when you train, tiny muscle tears occur and your muscles need time to repair themselves. It is better to weight train no more than two or three times per week. And, remember to always leave a day between your training sessions (but, stretching exercises can be done daily).

STRENGTHENING

Strengthening Guidelines (Arms & Legs)

- Always lift the weight in a slow and controlled fashion in both directions

- When exercising a muscle group, your goal is to fatigue or tire that muscle group. This means your muscle(s) will feel too tired to lift the weight even once more and you will need a rest

- For strength training, the weight or resistance is correct if your muscle is tired after one set of 8-12 repetitions of the exercise. Rest and repeat repetitions for one or two more sets

- For muscle endurance training, the weight or resistance is correct if your muscle is tired after one set of 20 repetitions of the exercise. Rest and repeat 20 repetitions for two more sets

- Exercises should not be painful while you perform them or cause excessive soreness afterwards

Note: Opinion varies on the need to repeat sets of repetitions in strength training. Some believe one set is adequate, so choose what is best for you.

SHOULDER ROTATION (Outward)

- Lying on your side, hold your top arm at the side of your body with your elbow bent at 90 degrees

- Holding a weight, start with your hand resting against the front of your body and slowly raise and lower your forearm while keeping your elbow fixed against your side

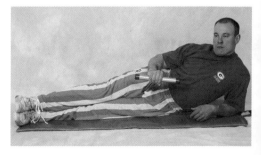

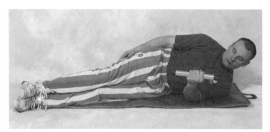

SHOULDER ROTATION (Inward)

- Lying on your side, hold your bottom arm slightly in front of your body with your elbow bent to 90 degrees. You can place a pillow under your head for comfort

- Holding a weight, start with your hand resting against the front of your body, slowly lower and raise your forearm keeping your elbow fixed against your body

The rotators of the shoulder can be exercised using a specialty rubber band.

FRONT SHOULDER LIFT

- With your arms at your sides, hold a weight in each hand

- Keeping your arm straight, slowly lift one arm at a time to shoulder level and lower back to your side

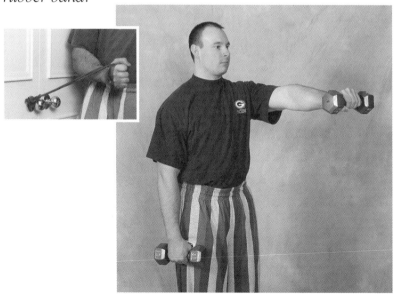

STRENGTHENING (cont'd)

SIDE SHOULDER LIFT

- With your arms at your sides, hold a weight in each hand
- While keeping your arms slightly bent, slowly lift both of your arms to your shoulder level and then lower them back to your sides

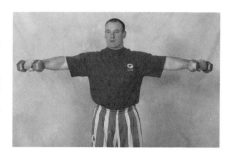

TWO HANDED FRONT SHOULDER LIFT

- Hold a single weight or barbell in front of your body with both hands

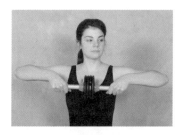

- Slowly bring the bar to your shoulder level by bending at your elbows and then lower the bar back to the original position

FRONT CHEST MUSCLES

- With a weight in each of your hands, lie flat or on an incline (each position works different parts of your muscles)
- Hold your arms with the weights straight out to your sides and level with your shoulders. Then, while keeping your arms slightly bent, slowly raise and lower the weights so that the weights meet directly above you

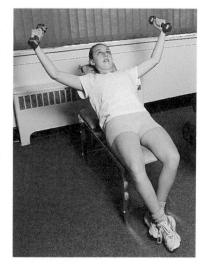

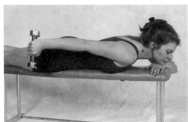

SHOULDER & UPPER BACK MUSCLES

- Lying face down on a bed or exercise table, hold a weight in your hand and hang your arm straight down with your palm facing inwards

- Keeping your arm straight, slowly raise your arm back behind you and then lower the weight to the starting position

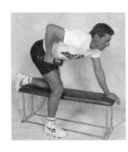

MID-BACK MUSCLES

- Support yourself with your knee and extended arm on a bench. With a weight in your hand, hang your arm straight down

- While keeping your back flat and shoulders level, slowly lift your arm straight upward by bending your elbow. Then slowly lower the weight back down

BICEPS

- Hold a weight in each hand, with your arms at your sides

- Moving one arm at a time, slowly bend your elbow with your palm facing upwards. Bring your weight towards your shoulder and then slowly lower it back to your side

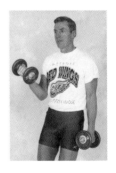

TRICEPS

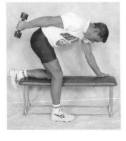

- Support yourself with your knee and extended arm on a bench

- With a weight in your hand, keep your upper arm in line with your body against your waistline

- From a bent elbow position slowly straighten your elbow and then slowly return it to the bent position

STRENGTHENING (cont'd)

SQUAT

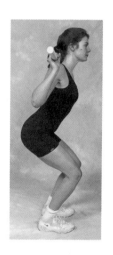

- Stand with your feet shoulder-width apart and your toes turned out slightly. For balance, you should hold your arms straight out in front of your body, or hold a bar/broomstick on either side as it sits behind your neck across your shoulders

- Slowly lower and raise your body. To do this correctly, bend your knees and push your buttocks out as though you are sitting back into a chair and the weight is in your heels. Only squat to the point you feel you are working your muscles but are still comfortable. For although your long-range goal should be to have your thighs parallel to the floor, few people ever achieve this

Controlled squats are a fast way to tone and strengthen your legs and hips.

STATIONARY STRAIGHT LINE LUNGE

- Take a big step forward with one foot while the toes of both of your feet point forward. Your front leg gets the workout, your back leg provides balance

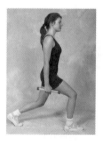

- For better balance, place your hands on your hips, hold a weight in each hand at your sides, or hold onto a stable object

- Slowly bend your hip and knee to lower your body. Keep your knee pointing forward and over your ankle but not in front of your ankle. Lunge or lower yourself to the point you feel you are working your muscles but are still comfortable. Slowly raise back up by pushing your heel into the floor

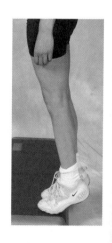

CALF MUSCLES

- While standing, slowly raise and lower your heels. This can be performed on a flat floor, or on a step to allow your heels to drop down lower than your toes (Skating is also a good workout for your calf muscles)

ABDOMINAL MUSCLES

Abdominal muscles play an important role in many of our daily activities. Stronger abdominals assist us with good posture; hold our internal organs in place; enhance our appearance; and provide the strength necessary to improve our technique and performance during sports activities. The oblique muscles of the abdomen are particularly important in golf.

The traditional sit-up is no longer recommended for it puts undue stress on your lower back. Abdominal crunches are now the exercises of choice, for these exercises minimize unnecessary movement to your back and maximize muscle work. You can safely exercise your abdominal muscles daily. Start with three sets of five repetitions and over the course of two weeks increase to three sets of 15 to 20 repetitions.

STRAIGHT ABDOMINALS

- Lie on your back with your knees bent and your feet flat

- Support your head with your fingertips and lift your head towards the ceiling so that your shoulder blades are just off the floor

- Hold this for two counts

Healthy Hints

- Always start and end each abdominal workout with ten 'sloppy' push-ups

- Do not pull your head or neck

- Perform five backward neck bends if you stress your neck

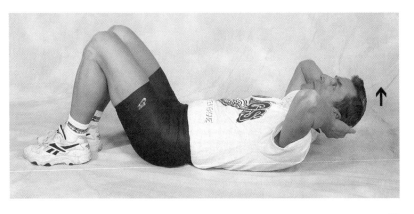

STRENGTHENING (cont'd)

OBLIQUE ABDOMINALS

• Lie down on your back with your knees bent and rest your left ankle on your right knee

• Support your head with your right hand, leave your left arm resting at your side

• Lift your right shoulder towards your left knee

• Hold this for two counts

After you complete your repetitions, do this to your other side

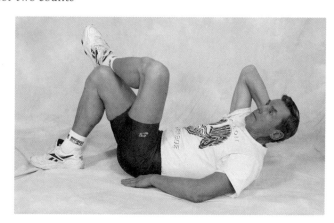

BACK MUSCLES

You have layers of varying lengths of back muscles that run from the base of your skull to the bottom of your spine. These muscles allow you to bend backwards, and the deeper, shorter muscles are important for rotation. When your back muscles are strong, bending forward and lifting will cause less strain. Trunk flexibility, combined with strong abdominals and back muscles, allow for smooth, strong trunk rotation during your golf swing.

When strengthening your back muscles, start with the easy back arch and progress to difficult. For endurance, increase your holding time and be sure to start with the easy back arch again. Work up to being able to hold the position for one minute.

EASY BACK ARCH

- Lie on your stomach with two pillows under your lower abdomen and anchor your feet

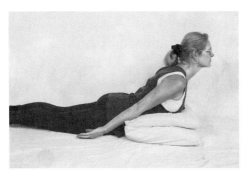

- With your arms at your sides, lift your upper body as high as you can while arching your back

- Hold this for five counts

Repeat this exercise five times

DIFFICULT BACK ARCH

- Lie on your stomach with two pillows under your lower abdomen and anchor your feet

- With your arms extended over your head, lift your upper body as high as you can while arching your back

- Hold this for five counts

Repeat this exercise five times

Trunk flexibility, combined with strong abdominals and back muscles, allow for smooth, strong trunk rotation during your golf swing.

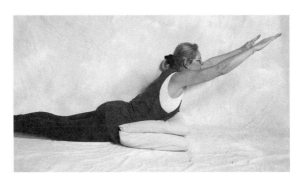

STRETCHING

We lose flexibility over time due to inactivity and poor habits. The imbalances associated with lost flexibility often lead to pain and interfere with our movement. And, tightness in your hips, trunk, upper limbs and neck can adversely affect your golf swing.

To improve or increase your flexibility, you should perform stretching exercises daily. Once you have regained your flexibility, stretching every other day will maintain your gains. Remember to warm up your muscles before you stretch (2-3 minutes). Stretching can be done anywhere, in your home, your office or at the gym.

Stretching Guidelines

- Move to the point where you feel a comfortable pull. If this pull lessens during the stretch, then stretch a little more. You should feel no pain

- For optimal results hold the stretch for 30 seconds. If for some reason you are unable to hold for 30 seconds, hold for a shorter period of time. Return to start position between each stretch

- Repeat each stretch three times in the same direction

- Repeat for the opposite side

NECK ROTATION STRETCH

- While sitting, place your left arm behind your back and lean against it

- With your right hand placed on the left side of your cheek or forehead, turn your head to the right to the point where you feel a comfortable pull

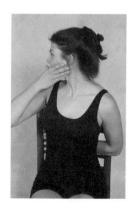

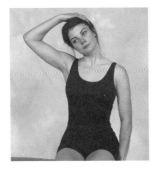

NECK SIDE BENDING STRETCH

- While sitting, place your left hand under your buttocks

- Grasp the top of your head with your right hand and tip your head to the right side to the point where you feel a comfortable pull

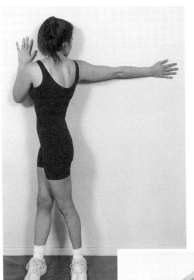

TRUNK ROTATION STRETCH
(Neck, Shoulder & Mid-back)

- Stand about one foot away from a wall with your back facing the wall. Place your feet a shoulders width apart and keep your legs straight

- Twist to the right until your upper body is facing the wall with your palms on the wall. Your left elbow is bent and your right elbow is straight. Pushing through your right hand increases the stretch

TRUNK SIDE BENDING STRETCH

- Kneel facing a wall and rest your arms above your head against the wall

- Slowly walk your arms and trunk to one side to the point where you feel a comfortable pull

STRETCHING (cont'd)

FULL SIDE STRETCH

- Cross your right leg over your left and get your balance. Interlace your fingers and raise your arms above your head with palms facing upwards

- Slowly bend your trunk to the left to the point where you feel a comfortable pull

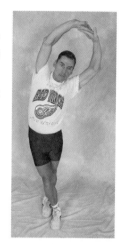

BACK OF SHOULDER & UPPER ARM STRETCH

- Place your left hand on your right shoulder

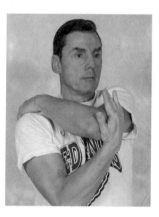

- Grasp your left elbow and move it across your body towards your right shoulder to the point where you feel a comfortable pull

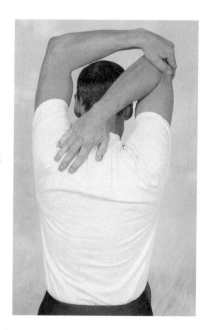

SHOULDER, UPPER ARM & SIDE STRETCH

- Place your right hand behind your left upper back

- Hold your right elbow with your left hand and move your elbow behind your head to the point where you feel a comfortable pull

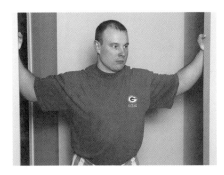

FRONT CHEST MUSCLES STRETCH

- Stand in a doorway and raise both of your arms out to the side with elbows bent to 90 degrees

- Rest your forearms on the sides of the doorway. Lean your body forward to the point where you feel a comfortable pull

GROIN STRETCH

- Sit on the floor, and bend your knees so the bottom of your feet touch

- Apply pressure to both inner knees stretching to the point where you feel a comfortable pull

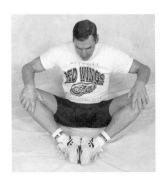

Note: A groin stretch can also be done lying on your back with your knees bent, bottoms of your feet together allowing your knees to drop out to the sides.

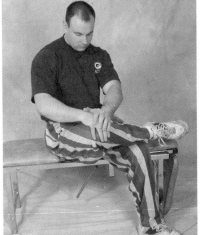

HIP ROTATOR STRETCH

- Place your right ankle on your left knee

- Apply downward pressure with your hands to the inside of the knee to the point where you feel a comfortable pull

STRETCHING (cont'd)

HIP ROTATOR /BUTTOCKS STRETCH

- While sitting, cross your right leg over your left

- With both hands, bring your right knee across and up towards your left shoulder to the point where you feel a comfortable pull

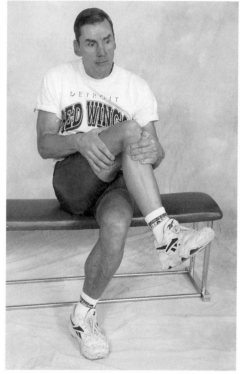

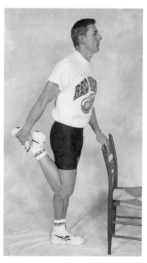

FRONT LEG STRETCH

- Place your hand on a stable surface for support

- Bend your leg, grasp your ankle/foot with your other hand and bring your foot towards your buttocks to the point where you feel a comfortable pull

BACK LEG STRETCH

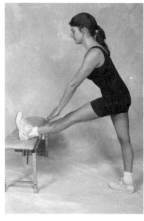

- Raise your leg and rest your heel on a stable surface while keeping your knee straight and your toes pointing to the ceiling

- Keeping your back straight, bend forward at the hip to the point where you feel a comfortable pull in the back of your leg (you can rest your hands on your thigh or reach towards your toe, be careful to not bend your back)

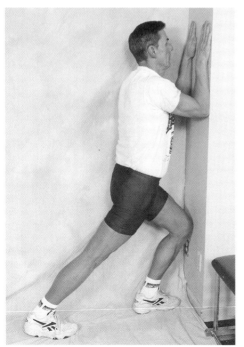

CALF STRETCH

- Stand back from a stable surface and take one long step forward to position your legs. Your front leg should be bent and your back leg straight. (You are stretching the back leg)

- Place your hands on the surface and move your hips forward to the point where you feel a comfortable pull. (Keep your back leg straight, heel flat and toes pointing forwards)

YEAR ROUND CONDITIONING

HEART & LUNG HEALTH

Aerobic exercises involve whole body activity. You use all of your large muscle groups when you walk, jog, or swim. Aerobic exercises are those that safely and comfortably increase your breathing and heart rates for extended periods of time without disturbing the balance between your intake and use of oxygen. Huffing and puffing after you exercise means this balance has been disturbed and you are paying back an oxygen debt. When you perform aerobic exercises correctly you are helping to improve this oxygen delivery system.

Choose an activity that you enjoy. It is not necessary to use equipment at a health club or gym. Walk your dog, do some gardening or maybe go for a bike ride. Start slowly, gradually increase the length of time of your chosen activity and eventually increase the intensity or how hard you work. Listen to your body and monitor your pulse. Get ready to feel good, have more energy, and last longer.

These steps should be followed when doing aerobic exercises:

1. RESTING HEART RATE
One of the first signs of improved aerobic fitness is a lower resting heart rate or pulse. Be sure to check your pulse regularly and monitor your improvement over time.

2. WARM-UP
A warm-up lasting three to five minutes prepares your body and muscles for your aerobic workout. Mimicking your chosen activity at an easy pace is a good way to warm up. This will increase the circulation to the muscles that you will soon be using more intensely.

3. TECHNIQUE

Perform your exercise at a steady, moderate pace. Pay attention to your posture and specific details related to your chosen activity. Use good technique.

4. INTENSITY

Studies suggest it is good to exercise within an "aerobic training zone." This means you work just hard enough to have your heart rate enter into your "Target Heart Rate Zone." If you work too hard, the ability of your heart and lungs to supply oxygen to your muscles becomes limited, for they can't keep up with the oxygen demand. Before you can establish your own target heart rate zone, you must calculate your "Predicted Maximal Heart Rate".

INDIVIDUAL TYPE	PREDICTED MAXIMAL HEART RATE CALCULATION	EXAMPLE 40 YEAR OLD
Women & Physically Inactive Men	220 minus your age	220 - 40 = 180 beats per minute
Conditioned, Physically Active Men	205 minus $\frac{1}{2}$ your age	205 - 20 = 185 beats per minute

The formula to calculate your Target Heart Rate Zone is 65-80% of your predicted maximal heart rate.

EXAMPLE:
Outlined below is an example for a 40 year woman or 40 year old physically inactive man with a predicted maximal heart rate of 180.

% RATE	TARGET HEART RATE ZONE	RANGE
65	180 x .65 = 117	lower end
80	180 x .80 = 144	upper end

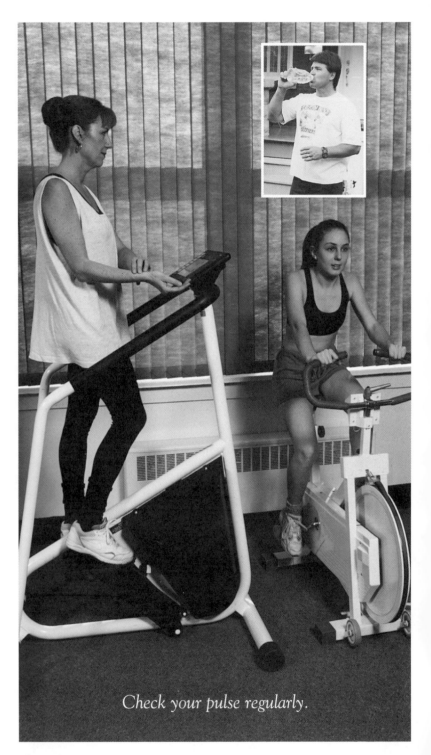

Check your pulse regularly.

HEART & LUNG HEALTH (cont'd)

Work your heart and lungs — and your heart and lungs will work for you.

5. MONITORING YOUR HEART RATE

You should monitor your heart rate to ensure you remain within your target training zone and to evaluate how long it takes your heart rate to recover after you cool down. Check your pulse just after your warm-up, twice during the aerobic component of your workout, and then after cool down. In time, you will recognize the feeling of working within your training zone. The 'talk test' is always a good check to use. As you exercise, you should be able to carry on a normal conversation without sounding out of breath.

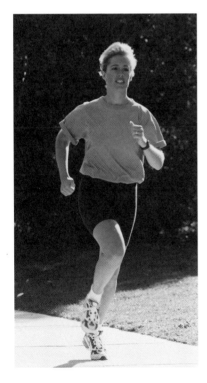

6. DURATION & FREQUENCY

The Institute for Aerobics Research recommends exercising for twenty minutes four times a week, or for thirty minutes three times a week.

7. COOL-DOWN

Never suddenly stop exercising. Your cool-down should take about five minutes and you should slow your exercise to a gradual stop. Your body needs to gradually return to its pre-exercise state.

8. FLUIDS

Drink water prior to, during and after exercise, thirst is not a reliable signal.

PRE-SEASON PREPARATION

You need to introduce golf-specific training into your conditioning program six to eight weeks prior to the start of every golf season. Year-round conditioning should include strengthening and stretching exercises that address the specific demands of the golf swing. But as the season approaches you should pick up a golf club and start some additional preparation to focus on your forearms, wrists and hands.

Although golf is not considered a strenuous sport, it produces a surprising number of injuries. The most commonly injured area in male golfers is the lower back. Female golfers are more prone to upper limb injuries, with wrist and hand pain the most common complaint. Wrist pain in female golfers is often caused by a poor grip (such as gripping the club too tightly) or poor technique. Be sure to have your golf professional check your swing and your grip.

Specific stretches for your wrists and thumbs and strengthening of your hand and forearm muscles will help prevent many problems involving the wrist, hand and elbow. These exercises can be performed in the comfort of your home. Remember, strong and flexible forearms, wrists and hands are all essential for good golf.

Tennis elbow is more common among golfers than golfer's elbow.

Stretching Guidelines

- Move to the point where you feel a comfortable pull. If this pull lessens during the stretch, then stretch a little more. You should feel no pain

- For optimal results hold the stretch for 30 seconds and repeat each stretch three times in the same direction

- Repeat for the opposite side

- Perform daily

THUMB STRETCH

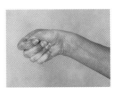

- Grasp your thumb in the palm of your hand with your fingers, thumb side facing the ceiling

- Keep your wrist in a neutral position, slowly tip your hand down to the floor to stretch

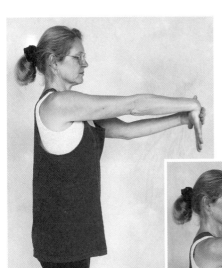

WRIST/FOREARM STRETCHES

- Hold your arm in front of you, keeping your elbow straight

- Point your fingers down to the floor; use your other hand to apply the stretch (Extensors)

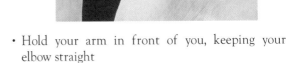

- Hold your arm in front of you, keeping your elbow straight

- Point your fingers up to the ceiling; use your other hand to apply the stretch (Flexors)

Strengthening Guidelines (Hands & Forearms)

- Always lift the weight in a slow and controlled fashion in both directions

- An ideal weight should allow you to perform three sets of ten repetitions. Rest between each set

- Exercises should not be painful while you perform them or cause excessive soreness afterwards

- Perform exercises three times a week allowing a day's rest in between

WRIST/FOREARM (Flexors)

- Rest your forearm on a firm surface with your hand and wrist extended over the edge and your palm facing the ceiling

- With a weight in your hand, raise and lower the weight ten times

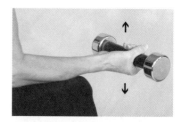

WRIST/FOREARM (Extensors)

- Rest your forearm on a firm surface with your hand and wrist extended over the edge and your palm facing the floor

- With a weight in your hand, raise and lower the weight ten times

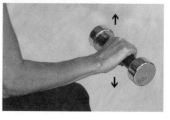

ELASTIC BAND EXERCISE

- Close your fingers and thumb together, place one to ten elastic bands around them (number depends on thickness of bands and on your strength)

- Slowly spread and release your fingers and thumb against the resistance of the bands

Items around the house such as a can of food or a book can be used as weights for your exercises.

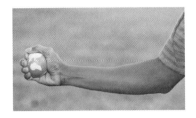

EXERCISE BALL SQUEEZE:

- Squeeze and release a tennis ball, squash ball or a resistance exercise ball to help strengthen your hands and forearms

You can do this anywhere, anytime.

ADVANCED FOREARM STRENGTHENING

- Tie a disk or other weight (bucket or purse) to a length of rope. Tie the other end to a piece of doweling

- With your arms held out in front of you slowly roll the dowel forward until the rope winds the weight to the top

- Reverse to roll the weight down again

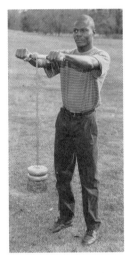

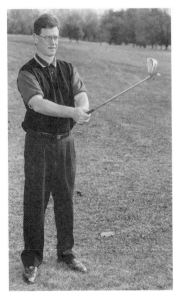

The following exercises involving golf clubs are ideal to further strengthen your muscles, improve your coordination and increase club control. Perform these two to four times a week.

CLUB CALLIGRAPHY

- Grip a short iron and lift the club to a point opposite your chest

- Slowly print your name in the air, accurately guiding the clubface

- Repeat until your muscles tire. You should not experience pain

PRE-SEASON PREPARATION

ONE-HANDED SWING

- Using a short iron, perform one-handed swings (always swing through and up to a full finish)

- If you are a right handed golfer, start with your left hand and repeat ten times

- Change hands and repeat five times (to strengthen weaker groups of muscles, maintain 2 to 1 ratio as you increase repetitions)

- Progress into one-handed shots

  (Left handed golfers should reverse this procedure)

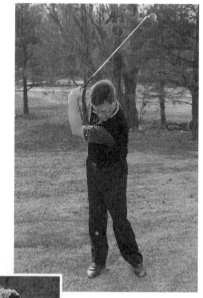

TWO-CLUB WORKOUT

- Using two irons, perform practice swings with a brief break between each swing

- Progress to continuous swings

FEET TOGETHER SWINGS

- With the ball teed and your feet together, practice hitting balls

- Start with a short iron and swing slowly, increase your pace once you gain a better sense of balance

- Once you can hit good shots consistently, try hitting shots with a longer iron and then with the ball on the turf

This encourages you to swing your arms and turn your body, rather than sway from side to side.

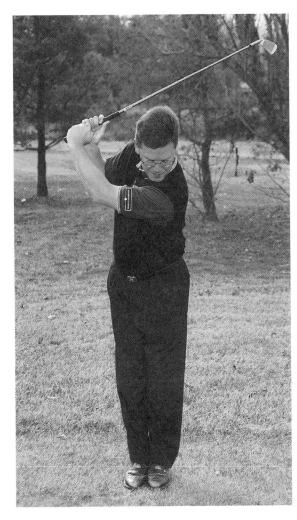

WARM-UP
& COOL-DOWN

WARM-UP

A warm-up prepares your body physically and mentally for your upcoming golf game. It also reduces the potential for injuries. And, the increased blood flow and flexibility with your warm-up improves muscle performance.

Allow approximately ten minutes to warm-up prior to the first tee or practicing on the driving range.

Start with a general warm-up exercise to get your blood flowing, such as climbing stairs, walking or jogging on the spot. Range of motion exercises or gentle stretches for the muscle groups used during the golf swing prepare your muscles for the game. Repeat each of these three times and do not hold positions more than a few counts. End your warm-up with practice swings, start with approximately half the power of your normal swing and gradually increase the power. The swing portion of your warm-up further prepares your muscles for the game and serves as a rehearsal for the first tee.

Start your warm-up by getting the blood flowing, climb stairs, walk or jog on the spot.

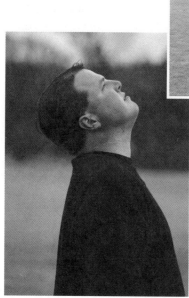

Protect your spine, perform five back bends and five backward neck bends.

FULL SIDE BEND

- Cross your right leg over your left and get your balance

- Interlace your fingers, raise your arms above your head with palms facing upwards

- Slowly bend your trunk to the left, return to your start position

Perform on both sides

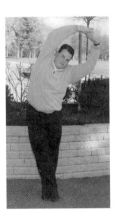

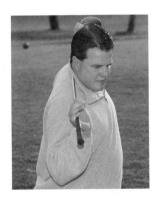

UPPER BODY ROTATION

- Stand straight, keep your hips level to the ground, place a club across your shoulders behind your head and hold each end of the club with your hands

- Slowly turn your shoulders to the right until you feel resistance, return to your start position

Perform in both directions

UPPER ARM & SHOULDER ELEVATION

- Place your hands widely apart on a towel and slowly raise the towel over the top of your head until you feel resistance, return to your start position

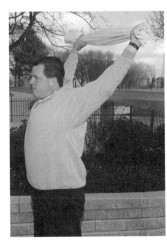

WARM-UP (cont'd)

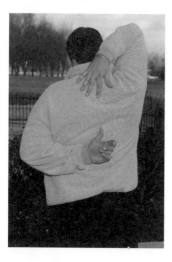

SHOULDER ROTATIONS

• Reach your right hand over your right shoulder and reach your left hand behind your back, try to touch fingertips

• Return to start position and repeat with opposite hands

DEEP KNEE BENDS

• Place your hand on your golf club or other stable surface for support

• Slowly perform deep knee bends

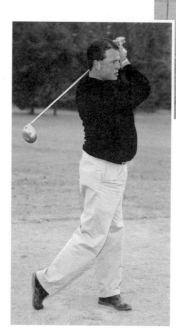

PRACTICE SWINGS

• Remember to start with approximately half the power of your normal swing and gradually increase the power

COOL-DOWN

Your cool-down consists of stretching exercises after the game to help increase flexibility and promote removal of waste products (lactic acid) from your muscles. This also helps to reduce your muscle soreness. Perform three of each stretch and hold the stretch for ten seconds (notice this is different from the 30-second stretches recommended for conditioning). To undo the effects of putting and eyeing the ball during your day on the course, perform five chin tucks before you start your stretches.

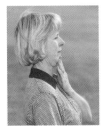

End your game with a cool-down.

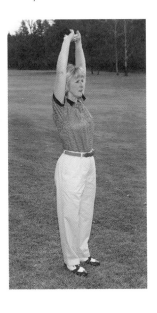

UPPER BODY STRETCH

- Standing tall, clasp your hands together and reach for the sky

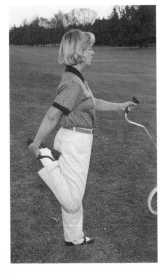

FRONT LEG STRETCH

- Place your hand on your golf cart or other stable surface for support

- Bend your leg, grasp your ankle/foot with your other hand and bring your foot towards your buttocks to the point where you feel a comfortable pull

Perform on both sides

59

COOL-DOWN (cont'd)

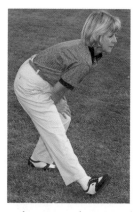

BACK LEG STRETCH

- Bend your left knee and place your hands on your thigh above your knee. Place your right heel on the ground ahead of you keeping your knee straight and your toes pointing to the sky

- Keep your back straight, lean your body forward by bending at the hips, to the point where you feel a comfortable pull

Perform on both sides

CHEST, HAND, ARM & SHOULDER STRETCH

- Lock your fingers together behind your back with your palms facing outwards

- Slowly straighten your elbows and lift your hands away from your body to the point where you feel a comfortable pull

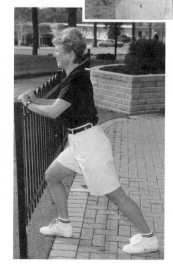

CALF STRETCH

- Stand back from a stable surface, take one long step forward to position your legs. Your front leg should be bent and your back leg straight. (You are stretching the back leg)

- Place your hands on the surface and move your hips forward to the point where you feel a comfortable pull. (Keep your back leg straight, heel flat and toes pointing forwards)

Perform on both sides

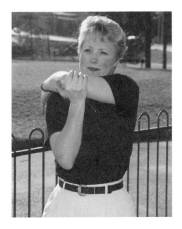

BACK OF SHOULDER & UPPER ARM STRETCH

- Place your left hand on your right shoulder

- Grasp your left elbow and move it across your body towards your right shoulder to the point where you feel a comfortable pull

Perform on both sides

SHOULDER, UPPER ARM & SIDE STRETCH

- Place your right hand behind your left upper back

- Hold your right elbow with your left hand and move your elbow behind your head to the point where you feel a comfortable pull

Perform on both sides

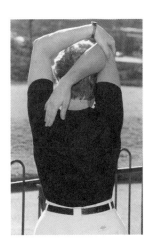

Massaging sore spots in a muscle can help prevent problems. Listen to your body.

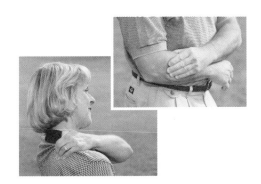

PROTECTION & HYDRATION — THE ELEMENTS

Golf is a wonderful way to enjoy the great outdoors. But with most courses having little shade and a lot of direct sunlight, you need to protect yourself from the elements.

Sun can burn your skin, damage the retina of your eyes and contribute to cataracts. Prolonged exposure to the sun can also result in skin cancer. Protecting yourself can be as simple as putting on sunscreen, wearing a hat or covering up. Ultraviolet protective sunglasses can also greatly reduce the damage to your eyes.

Spending time outside on hot, humid days can cause heat stress. The first symptoms are headaches, dizziness, fatigue and weakness. If you develop any of these, loosen your clothing, rest in a cool area and drink plenty of water.

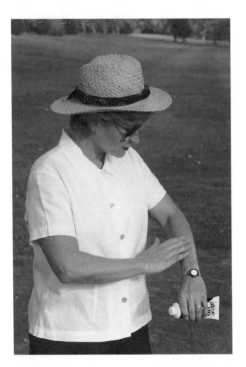

Healthy Hints

- Always apply sunscreen with a sun protection factor (SPF) of 15 or greater. Apply prior to arriving at the course and reapply sunscreen throughout the day

- Drink water before, during and after your game

- Wear a hat, preferably one with a brim

- Wear sunglasses

- Avoid long periods of exposure to the sun between 11 a.m and 4 p.m.

- Use an umbrella, or seek the shade of trees whenever possible

PROTECTION & HYDRATION — THE ELEMENTS

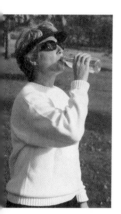

Water is critical to the healthy functioning of almost every cell in our bodies. We lose a lot of water during a typical day, and even more when we are active or active in warm or hot conditions. Always have water available to drink prior to, during and after your golf game.

If you are playing on a course away from home, in unfamiliar territory, be sure to inquire about local vegetation, insects and other wildlife.

With people spending more time outdoors, the overall number of lightning deaths is expected to increase. Lightning normally strikes the tallest object in its range, and a person standing in the middle of an open field is a target. The Lightning Safety Group, appointed by the American Meteorological Society in 1998, advises people to avoid being near high places, open fields, isolated trees and bodies of water. You will notice these criteria fit many golf courses. Don't take chances. Do not take refuge in your golf cart — head for the clubhouse. If you can see lightning or hear thunder, you are already at risk. In the United States, lightning is responsible for five to ten deaths per year and more than 100 injuries on the golf course alone. Be safe!

Protecting your eyes with sunglasses today may mean seeing the golf ball tomorrow.

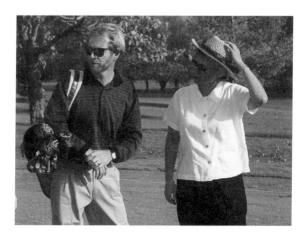

STANDING

When standing for a long time, the muscles that support your body get tired and lazy. Your natural low-back hollow becomes excessive. This can result in a 'sway back' over time. Young teenagers, particularly if they're tall, can feel awkward amongst their peers. As a result they often slouch in an attempt to go unnoticed and develop poor posture habits. Remind them to stand upright, just like the army commands from old movies: "Stand Tall, Chest Up and Stomach In!"

We all stand bent over for many activities: children at craft tables, teenagers over microscopes, parents at the kitchen counter and golfers lining up a putt. Whenever you do things that have you bent forward for long periods of time, give your back a regular stretch break and do five back bends.

Always interrupt activities that require you to stand bent forward. Do back bends.

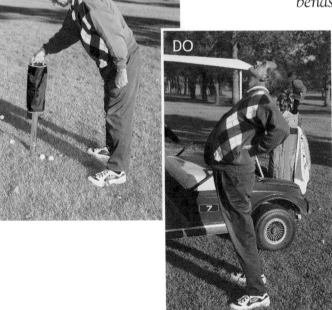

DO

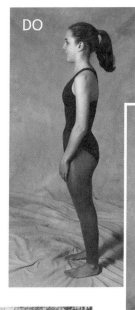

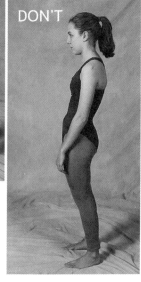

Healthy Hints

When standing for long periods:

- Occasionally shift your weight from one foot to the other

- Raise one foot and rest it on an elevated surface such as your golf bag

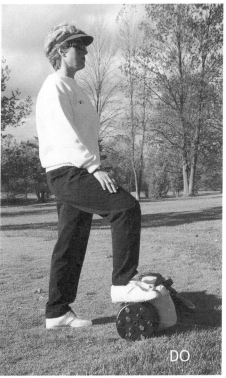

It is not uncommon to spend four and five hours on the golf course at one time. The prolonged standing associated with this can lead to fatigue and aching across the lower back area. You can temporarily relieve this back strain by raising one foot and resting it on your golf bag or golf cart.

TEEING, RETRIEVING & LIFTING

BODY BASICS

If your work day routinely involves repeated lifting, standing in a bent forward position or prolonged sitting; bending to tee or retrieve the golf ball may be the movement that triggers a bout of debilitating back pain. Healthy habits need to be part of your daily routines, including your day at the golf course. Remember to bend your knees, retain the hollow in your lower back and crouch down when teeing the ball or picking it up.

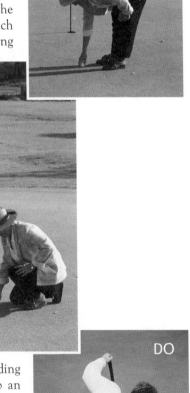

DON'T

DO

DO

If you carry your golf bag, proper body mechanics is a must! As young children we have the right idea. Watch your children pick up a toy or a crayon from the floor. Children bend both knees and crouch to pick up the object, whether it is large or small, heavy or light. But, as children grow older, they develop the poor lifting and 'picking up' habits that are so often seen in adults. Bending forward from your waist to pick up an object, lifting an object that is far away from your body, or twisting while you lift, are all bad habits.

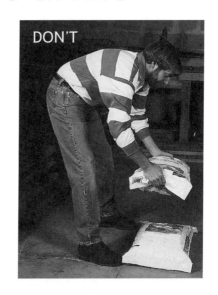

DON'T

As children grow older, they develop the poor lifting and 'picking up' habits so often seen in adults.

Healthy Hints

- Do five back bends prior to lifting

- Stand close to the load

- Retain the hollow in your lower back

- Bend your knees and drop down to the load

- Hold the load close to your body

- Lift the load by straightening your knees

- When standing, shift your feet to avoid twisting

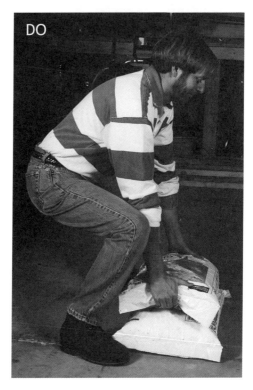

DO

GOLF BAGS & BEYOND

Whether you choose to use a golf cart, a riding cart or carry your clubs, golfing involves lifting and carrying your golf bag many times. Sitting as you drive to the golf course and then lifting your clubs out of the trunk puts you at risk for back pain. Using a lower-back roll or a full-back support while you sit, and performing back bends before you lift, will help prevent problems. If possible, put your clubs in the back seat of your car, so that you can position yourself better when you lift them.

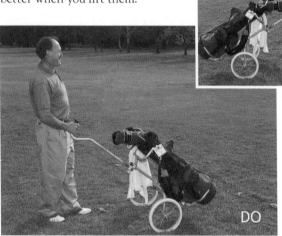

Healthy Hints

- A light bag is safer to carry

- If you use a one-strap system, be sure to alternate the side you carry your golf bag on

- A two-strap system helps to distribute the weight more evenly across your shoulders

- If walking long distances with a heavy bag, stop and take a break. Don't wait for pain!

- Push a wheeled golf cart rather than pulling it

- If using a motorized golf cart, try to sit in an upright position. If you have back problems, consider using a full-back support

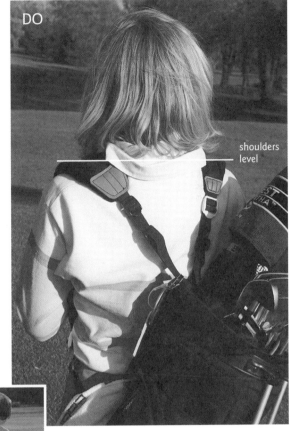

DO

shoulders level

The average golf bag weighs 22 pounds. Imagine carrying that many groceries around a four-mile golf course in a day.

DON'T

shoulders tilted

If you choose to carry your golf bag, consider the recently introduced two-strap system. This system helps to distribute the weight more evenly (much like a backpack) and allows you to maintain good posture. Two-strap systems are available at most pro shops and golf stores.

GOLF BAGS & BEYOND

PURSES & WALLETS

Most women carry a purse every day. Purses should be light and tucked under the arm. Shoulder straps should be worn across the body, rather than hung from one side. Carrying a heavy purse over your shoulder can lead to many physical complaints. More recently, I have been using a fanny pack or a small, light purse with the shoulder strap across my body. Both work well, but the biggest challenge is to reduce the load in your purse!

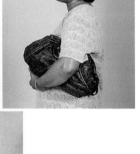

DO

Carrying your wallet in your same back pocket may be convenient but can alter your posture and lead to back problems later in life.

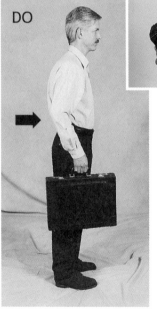

DO

BRIEFCASES & CARRYBAGS

If you can't keep your elbow slightly bent when you carry a bag, then it is too heavy.

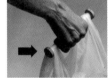

CARRY BAG HANDLE

Healthy Hints

- Use a small purse or fanny pack
- Carry your purse tucked under your arm and be sure to alternate the side you carry it on
- Keep your elbows slightly bent when carrying briefcases, suitcases and groceries
- Use a carry bag handle to protect your joints

GOLFER'S FEET

Whether your sport is golf, squash, or a walk in the park, you need your feet to keep you going. When we are young, we tend to take our feet for granted and we wear poorly designed shoes and often wear the same shoes for every sports activity — regardless of the physical demands to our feet. And then there is the high heel shoe, which challenges not only the foot but also body alignment.

Select your shoes carefully, our feet start to change in our early 40's making our feet more prone to pain.

When golfing, you may be on your feet for four to five hours so comfortable and supportive shoes are important.

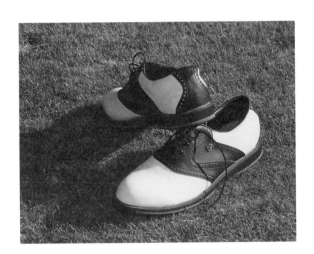

Healthy Hints

- Break in new shoes slowly and carry a back-up pair with you to change into

- Give yourself a foot massage after a long day on the course

- If foot pain persists, seek advice from a health professional

- Good golf shoes won't do the trick if you are careless with your everyday footwear

- Take a break, give your feet a rest

RELAXING AT THE 19TH HOLE

Think of what you do after a full day of golf—you probably relax. You may sit in the clubhouse for a drink or you may sit outside continuing to enjoy the fresh air. And at some point you will also end up sitting for the drive home. And it is probably safe to say sitting posture is not at the forefront of your thoughts when you do these things.

Many golfers experience back pain after a day of golf and most attribute their pain to golfing, even though their pain did not begin until after they slouched for an hour or two, chatting with friends. Your spine is more vulnerable to problems after every sports activity. Some simple steps can help you avoid this.

Perform five back bends and five chin tucks after the game and sit with good posture. A lower back roll or a rolled up towel supporting the inward curve in your lower back will help. And don't forget, when you are drinking, to make sure you bring your drink to your mouth rather than poking your head forward to your glass. Good posture is not hard to develop but it does take practice.

DO

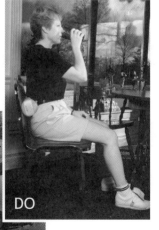

DO

DON'T

Healthy Hints

- Perform five back bends and five chin tucks after every sports activity, including golf

- Pay attention to your posture when relaxing after a workout. If you're sitting, maintain your natural inward curves in your neck and back

- Use a lower back roll as often as possible

72

RESTING

MATTRESS

The comfort and support given by a mattress is affected by the base it is placed on. It is best to place a mattress on a box spring of similar quality. If you will be placing it on a solid base, try it out before you buy it by placing it on the floor to check for comfort and support. Avoid mattresses that sag or are too hard.

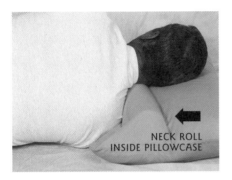

NECK ROLL
INSIDE PILLOWCASE

PILLOWS

Remember one pillow is enough! Since your pillow should support your head and neck, the pillow needs only to fill the hollow between your head and shoulders. Feather or foam chip pillows work well since you can adjust their shape to support your neck.

Neck rolls provide support to those who have difficulty getting adequate support from a pillow. The roll is best placed inside the pillowcase.

Care for your spine off the course and it will treat you well on the course.

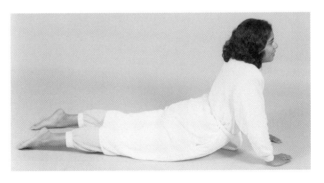

Healthy Hints

• Use one pillow to sleep or try a neck roll inside your pillowcase if you need better support

• Do five chin tucks when you wake up

• Do five 'sloppy' push-ups when you wake up

HEALTHY HABITS ON THE GOLF COURSE

Adults spend a great deal of time at the golf course, and our young people have started to spend more time there as well. This summary has been compiled as an easy reference for everyone.

- Maintain the inward curve in your lower back when sitting in the car, golf cart or clubhouse

- Interrupt long periods of sitting. Do five back bends every sixty minutes

- Always warm up and cool down

- Wear a hat and ultraviolet protective sunglasses

- Carry your golf bag over both shoulders and walk upright. If you have a one strap system, alternate sides and walk upright

- When lifting, bend your knees, keep your back straight, hold your golf bag close and do not twist your body

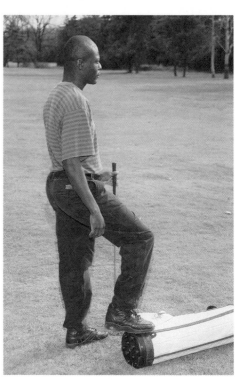

- Push your golf cart, don't pull

- Stand tall when standing for long periods, and occasionally shift your weight from one foot to the other, or rest one foot on your golf bag or golf cart

- After each green, do a few chin tucks and one backward neck bend to counter eyeing the ball and putting

- After putting, do a few back bends if you feel a strain in your lower back

- When teeing or retrieving your golf ball, bend your knees and crouch down to the ball

- Carry a water bottle and a healthy snack in your golf bag

- Apply sunscreen throughout the day

- Take a shade break on hot, humid days

- Stop and stretch, don't wait for pain

Your goal should be to learn and practice healthy habits that will last a lifetime.

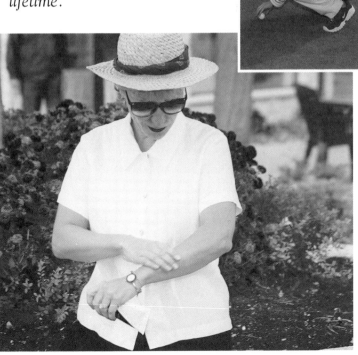

EVERYDAY LIVING CHECKLIST

This final checklist summarizes the key messages about everyday living found throughout **Body Basics** *fore golfers*. For what you do off the golf course affects how you feel and what you do on the golf course.

- Start and end your day with five 'sloppy' push-ups and five chin tucks

- Sit with an inward curve in your lower back

- Be active everyday

- Drink water before, during and after physical activity

- Warm up, cool down, and use good technique every time you exercise

- Play hard for thirty minutes three times a week or twenty minutes four times a week

- Always exercise prior to eating

- Do five back bends after all strenuous workouts

- Do ten 'sloppy' push-ups before and after each abdominal workout

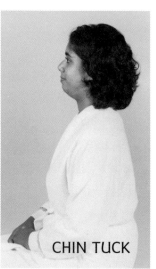

CHIN TUCK

- Walking, jogging and weight training strengthens bones

- Eat healthy foods. Limit fatty foods and sweets

- When standing for long periods, stand tall and occasionally shift your weight from one foot to the other

- When lifting, bend your knees, keep your back straight, hold the object close and do not twist your body

- Try to bend backward as you sneeze or cough to protect your spine

- Keep your elbow slightly bent when carrying a bag

- Use a carry bag handle when appropriate

- Interrupt long periods of sitting. Do five back bends every sixty minutes

- Interrupt long periods of deskwork. Do five chin tucks every sixty minutes

- Take stretch breaks every sixty minutes when doing repetitive activities

- Be good to your eyes, look up and focus further away every now and then or if you feel eye strain

- When working at a computer, remember to:

    - maintain the inward curve of your back and hold your head upright

    - keep arms at your side, elbows at 90° and your forearms and wrists parallel to the floor

    - sit with the monitor an arm's length away

- Use only one pillow to sleep

- Remember, year round conditioning helps you stay healthy, pain-free and injury free

- Pre-season preparation should start one to two months prior to your first game

- Always practice healthy habits on the golf course

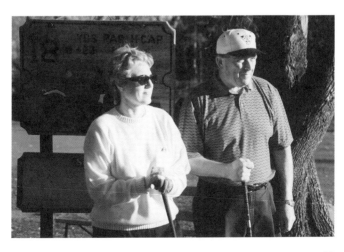

BIBLIOGRAPHY

BOOKS

1. Amen, Karen, *The Crunch*, London, Vermillion, 1994.
2. Anderson, Bob, *Stretching at your computer or desk*, California, Shelter Publications, 1997.
3. Anderson, Bob; Burke, Ed; Pearl, Bill; *Getting in Shape: Workout Programs For Men & Women*; California, Shelter Publications; New York: Random House, 1994.
4. Chalmers Mill, Wendy, *Repetitive Strain Injury*, London, Thorsons, 1994.
5. Conwell, Timothy, *Golfercise: The Golf Fitness Manual*, Colorado, Peak Performance Publications, 1996.
6. Cooper, Robert K., *Health & Fitness Excellence: The Scientific Action Plan*, Boston, Houghton Mifflin, 1989.
7. Fine, Judylaine, *The Ultimate Back Book: Understand, Manage, and Conquer Your Back Pain*, Toronto, Stoddart, 1997.
8. Merris, Eddie; McTeigue, Michael; *Golf For The Young*, Los Angeles, Los Angeles School District, 1981.
9. McLean, Jim, *Golf Digest's Book of Drills*, Connecticut, NYT Special Services Inc., A New York Times Company, 1990.
10. McIlwain, Harris, *Osteoporosis*, Prevention Management, Treatment, New York, Toronto: Wiley, 1988.
11. McKenzie, Robin, *Treat Your Own Back*, Spinal Publications Ltd., New Zealand, 1985.
12. McKenzie, Robin, *Treat Your Own Neck*, Spinal Publications Ltd., New Zealand, 1983.
13. Nelson, Miriam, Ph.D., *Strong Women Stay Young*; New York, Toronto, Bantam Books, 1997.
14. Roberts, Scott, *Fitness Walking*, Indianapolis, Masters Press, 1995.
15. Stirling, John, *Fit for Golf*, London, England, John Stirling, Alan Maryon-Davis, 1984.
16. Watson, Tom; Seitz, Nick; *Getting Back To Basics*, Connecticut, Golf Digest/Tennis, Inc., A New York Times Company, 1992.
17. Webb, Karen, *Body Basics for life: Simple steps to a healthy, pain-free you!*, Stratford, Ontario, Birchcliff Publishing Inc., 1998.

JOURNALS

1. Jobe, F.W., Moynes, D.R., Antonelli, D.J., 1986, *Rotator cuff function during a golf swing*, Am J Sports Med, 14:388-392.
2. Nesbitt, Lloyd, 'let your feet do the walking', the Health Journal, Canada's Authoritative Health Forum, Summer 1998.
3. Osteoporosis Society of Canada, 'Physical Activity Fact Sheet Series', Number 2.
4. Pink, M., Jobe, F.W., Perry, J., 1990, *Electromyographic analysis of the shoulder during the golf swing*, Am J Sports Med, 18(2):137-140.
5. Steinburg, Bill, 'Danger Zone: Timing and precautions help avoid burning rays of the sun', Golf Canada, June/July 1997.
6. Tant, Lisa, ' What's new under the sun ', Chatelaine, July 1998.

MAIL ORDERS

THE PERFECT GIFT THAT SHOWS YOU CARE!

For orders of 5 to 10 books, we'll pay the shipping costs to one address. Just fill out the order form below:

Name
_____

Address
_____

City _____ Province/State _____

Postal/Zip Code _____ Phone _____

MAIL this form along with your payment to:

BIRCHCLIFF PUBLISHING INC.
Suite 126
59 Albert Street
Stratford,
Ontario Canada
N5A 3K2

For more information
CALL:
(519) 273-3334 or
1-888-472-9121 or

FAX:
(519) 273-7222

Please send me _____ copies of **Body Basics** *fore golfers* @ $9.95 each	$
Please send me _____ copies of **Body Basics** *for life* @ $9.95 each	$
Postage & handling $1 per book Orders of 5 to 10 books = No Charge	$
SUBTOTAL	$
Add 7% GST (70¢ per book) Canadian Residents	$
TOTAL AMOUNT ENCLOSED	$

Please make cheque or money order payable to Birchcliff Publishing Inc.

An aggressive discount schedule is available for large volume orders.

- -

GIFT GIVING MADE EASY!

We will send a personally autographed **Body Basics** book directly to the recipient of your choice. Enclose a personal note or card and we will include it with your order.

Please send **Body Basics** ☐ *fore golfers* ☐ *for life* to:

Name
_____

Address
_____

City _____ Province/State _____

Postal/Zip Code _____

THE PERFECT GIFT THAT SHOWS YOU CARE!

Body Basics *fore golfers, Stay in the game, avoid pain!*, second in the **Body Basics** series, makes a great gift for golfers of all ages and playing abilities. A book filled with practical information for everyone. Check your local bookstore or order directly from us.

TO COMPLEMENT BODY BASICS *fore golfers...*

Simple and healthy products, as featured in this and other **Body Basics** *for life* books, are available through Birchcliff Publishing Inc. These convenient and inexpensive products are designed to relieve and prevent pain.

LOWER BACK ROLL

LOWER BACK ROLL: supports your natural inward curve and improves your posture. Lightweight and portable – ideal for your home, office and car.

NECK ROLL

NECK ROLL: supports your neck, improves your posture and enhances your sleep. Lightweight and portable. Fits easily inside your pillowcase.

CARRY BAG HANDLE

CARRY BAG HANDLE: holds one or more plastic, cloth or string bags safely. Protects your joints and muscles. Fits easily into your pocket or purse.

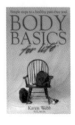

BODY BASICS *for life*: the first book in the **Body Basics** series provides readers with simple steps to a healthy pain-free life. Beautifully illustrated and suitable for all ages, it identifies poor body habits and clearly demonstrates how to change them.

All items are priced separately or conveniently packaged with books. Quantity discounts also available. For more information or to order by mail call toll free:

1-888-472-9121